Food Log Journal

TRACK YOUR FOOD. CHANGE YOUR LIFE.

Renata Trebing

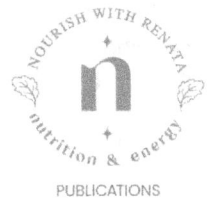

PUBLICATIONS

Food Log Journal: Track Your Food. Change Your Life.
Published by Nourish with Renata Publications
Houston, Texas
USA

www.nourishwithrenata.com

Contact publisher for bulk orders and permission requests.

Copyright © 2021 by Renata Trebing

Cover and interior book design & formatting by
Leesa Ellis of 3 ferns books ⟶ **www.3fernsbooks.com**

All rights reserved. No part of this publication may be reproduced, distributed, or transmitted in any form or by any means, including photocopying, recording, or other electronic or mechanical methods, without the prior written permission of the publisher, except in the case of brief quotations embodied in critical reviews and certain other noncommercial uses permitted by copyright law.

Printed in the United States of America.

ISBN: 978-0-578-94205-6

Introduction

One of the things I always say to my clients, and something that I shared in my cookbook, *Nourish Your Body,* is **"Listen to your body."**

I firmly believe that our bodies are giving us clues all the time about the foods that it needs to really thrive. All we have to do is listen.

But with the hustle and bustle of daily life, work, family, cleaning, laundry etc., it's easy for us to ignore the sounds of these clues.

So how do we stop ignoring and start to get back to hearing these body clues again?

Use a Food Log!

A Food Log is a great way to easily reflect back on the foods you eat and how your body feels. That's what this book is for.

For each drink, snack or meal, you can use this Food Log to write down what you ate. Then reflect back, or take a pause from your day, and note how your body felt after you ate or drank. For example, did you feel full, energized, focused and/or healthy? Or did you feel bloated, lethargic, guilty, and/or have a stomach upset? It is important to write down the physical, mental and emotional responses to the food too because there is a huge emotional component to food. This is what shapes our relationships with food from a young age until this very moment. Once we understand what that relationship is, we can then decide if we like that relationship or if we want to change it.

The same goes for the food we eat. Once you've logged your food for at least a few weeks, you will be able to see a trend in the foods that you eat and how your body responds to it. You can then keep this in mind whenever you are choosing what to eat for your next meal. You can decide if you are ok with eating that food because you know how you will feel after you eat it.

Understanding your body clues and how your body responds to different foods is why I love Food Logs. And that is why I wanted to share this convenient travel-sized Food Log with you. Take it

with you during the day and start creating the habit of writing in your Food Log after every meal.

If you use your Food Log but are unsure of how to analyze the information you wrote, feel free to let me know. You can reach out to me on social media **@nourish_with_renata** on Instagram to set up a Discovery Call and chat about your nutrition.

Make the decision today to start listening to your body. Start using your Food Log today!

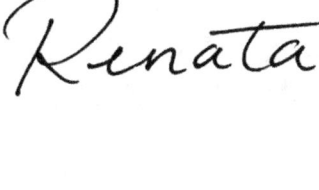

What I ate or drank

How I felt, physically & emotionally, after having it

What I ate or drank

How I felt, physically & emotionally, after having it

What I ate or drank

How I felt, physically & emotionally, after having it

Date: ___ / ___ / ___

What I ate or drank

How I felt, physically & emotionally, after having it

What I ate or drank

How I felt, physically & emotionally, after having it

What I ate or drank

How I felt, physically & emotionally, after having it

Date: ____ / ____ / ____

What I ate or drank

How I felt, physically & emotionally, after having it

What I ate or drank

How I felt, physically & emotionally, after having it

What I ate or drank

How I felt, physically & emotionally, after having it

Date: ___/___/___

What I ate or drank

How I felt, physically & emotionally, after having it

What I ate or drank

How I felt, physically & emotionally, after having it

What I ate or drank

How I felt, physically & emotionally, after having it

Date: ____ / ____ / ____

What I ate or drank

How I felt, physically & emotionally, after having it

What I ate or drank

How I felt, physically & emotionally, after having it

What I ate or drank

How I felt, physically & emotionally, after having it

Date: ___ / ___ / ___

What I ate or drank

How I felt, physically & emotionally, after having it

What I ate or drank

How I felt, physically & emotionally, after having it

What I ate or drank

How I felt, physically & emotionally, after having it

Date: ____ / ____ / ____

What I ate or drank

How I felt, physically & emotionally, after having it

What I ate or drank

How I felt, physically & emotionally, after having it

What I ate or drank

How I felt, physically & emotionally, after having it

Date: ___ / ___ / ___

What I ate or drank

How I felt, physically & emotionally, after having it

What I ate or drank

How I felt, physically & emotionally, after having it

What I ate or drank

How I felt, physically & emotionally, after having it

Date: ___ / ___ / ___

TIP #1
Are you eating enough protein?

Protein is an essential nutrient and helps us feel fuller for longer. It's also vital for ensuring our muscle fibers repair thicker and stronger, and can help us have more sustained energy all day. Aim to have a source of protein at every meal, roughly the size of your palm. Remember, protein can come from both animal sources and plant sources, so keep mixing it up and having lots of variety in your protein sources!

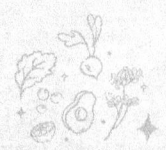

What I ate or drank

How I felt, physically & emotionally, after having it

What I ate or drank

How I felt, physically & emotionally, after having it

What I ate or drank

How I felt, physically & emotionally, after having it

Date: ____ / ____ / ____

What I ate or drank

How I felt, physically & emotionally, after having it

What I ate or drank

How I felt, physically & emotionally, after having it

What I ate or drank

How I felt, physically & emotionally, after having it

Date: ___ / ___ / ___

What I ate or drank

How I felt, physically & emotionally, after having it

What I ate or drank

How I felt, physically & emotionally, after having it

What I ate or drank

How I felt, physically & emotionally, after having it

Date: ___ / ___ / ___

What I ate or drank

How I felt, physically & emotionally, after having it

What I ate or drank

How I felt, physically & emotionally, after having it

What I ate or drank

How I felt, physically & emotionally, after having it

Date: ___ / ___ / ___

What I ate or drank

How I felt, physically & emotionally, after having it

What I ate or drank

How I felt, physically & emotionally, after having it

What I ate or drank

How I felt, physically & emotionally, after having it

Date: ____ / ____ / ____

What I ate or drank

How I felt, physically & emotionally, after having it

What I ate or drank

How I felt, physically & emotionally, after having it

What I ate or drank

How I felt, physically & emotionally, after having it

Date: ___ / ___ / ___

What I ate or drank

How I felt, physically & emotionally, after having it

What I ate or drank

How I felt, physically & emotionally, after having it

What I ate or drank

How I felt, physically & emotionally, after having it

Date: ____ / ____ / ____

TIP #2
Don't be scared of fat!

The word "fat" can often strike fear in the hearts of even the healthiest eater! But don't fear! Healthy fats are incredibly important. They help to slow down digestion which helps you feel full. We also need healthy fats to help with energy, to support cell growth and it helps you absorb certain vitamins and minerals. Healthy fats come from foods like avocado, nuts, seeds and coconut oil. Make sure they are a part of every meal!

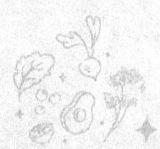

What I ate or drank

How I felt, physically & emotionally, after having it

What I ate or drank

How I felt, physically & emotionally, after having it

What I ate or drank

How I felt, physically & emotionally, after having it

Date: ____ / ____ / ____

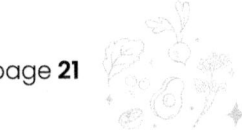

What I ate or drank

How I felt, physically & emotionally, after having it

What I ate or drank

How I felt, physically & emotionally, after having it

What I ate or drank

How I felt, physically & emotionally, after having it

Date: ___ / ___ / ___

What I ate or drank

_____

How I felt, physically & emotionally, after having it

_____

_____

What I ate or drank

_____

How I felt, physically & emotionally, after having it

_____

_____

What I ate or drank

_____

How I felt, physically & emotionally, after having it

_____

_____

Date: _____ / _____ / _____

What I ate or drank

How I felt, physically & emotionally, after having it

What I ate or drank

How I felt, physically & emotionally, after having it

What I ate or drank

How I felt, physically & emotionally, after having it

Date: ___ / ___ / ___

What I ate or drank

How I felt, physically & emotionally, after having it

What I ate or drank

How I felt, physically & emotionally, after having it

What I ate or drank

How I felt, physically & emotionally, after having it

Date: ___ / ___ / ___

What I ate or drank

How I felt, physically & emotionally, after having it

What I ate or drank

How I felt, physically & emotionally, after having it

What I ate or drank

How I felt, physically & emotionally, after having it

Date: ___ / ___ / ___

What I ate or drank

How I felt, physically & emotionally, after having it

What I ate or drank

How I felt, physically & emotionally, after having it

What I ate or drank

How I felt, physically & emotionally, after having it

Date: ___ / ___ / ___

TIP #3

Carbohydrates don't just exist in bread, pasta and pizza.

They are also in some very healthy and nutritious foods like fruits and vegetables. Reducing your refined carbohydrate intake can be beneficial for reducing inflammation and improving your gut health, but I am still a firm believer in having a broad range of colorful produce every day. This helps you have a multitude of vitamins and minerals, as well as lots of different sources of prebiotics, or fiber, in your eating plan.

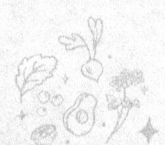

What I ate or drank

How I felt, physically & emotionally, after having it

What I ate or drank

How I felt, physically & emotionally, after having it

What I ate or drank

How I felt, physically & emotionally, after having it

Date: ___ / ___ / ___

What I ate or drank

How I felt, physically & emotionally, after having it

What I ate or drank

How I felt, physically & emotionally, after having it

What I ate or drank

How I felt, physically & emotionally, after having it

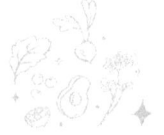

Date: ___ / ___ / ___

What I ate or drank

How I felt, physically & emotionally, after having it

What I ate or drank

How I felt, physically & emotionally, after having it

What I ate or drank

How I felt, physically & emotionally, after having it

Date: ___ / ___ / ___

What I ate or drank

How I felt, physically & emotionally, after having it

What I ate or drank

How I felt, physically & emotionally, after having it

What I ate or drank

How I felt, physically & emotionally, after having it

Date: ___ / ___ / ___

What I ate or drank

How I felt, physically & emotionally, after having it

What I ate or drank

How I felt, physically & emotionally, after having it

What I ate or drank

How I felt, physically & emotionally, after having it

Date: ___ / ___ / ___

What I ate or drank

How I felt, physically & emotionally, after having it

What I ate or drank

How I felt, physically & emotionally, after having it

What I ate or drank

How I felt, physically & emotionally, after having it

Date: ___ / ___ / ___

What I ate or drank

How I felt, physically & emotionally, after having it

What I ate or drank

How I felt, physically & emotionally, after having it

What I ate or drank

How I felt, physically & emotionally, after having it

Date: ___ / ___ / ___

TIP #4
Drink your water!

Most people are not drinking enough water each day. We reach for coffee or tea to get us moving in the morning, grab a sugary soda for lunch and then a glass of wine with dinner. But water is really what the body needs to ensure all body functions are working properly. We know that even a 1% reduction in hydration starts to impact your mental cognition, so imagine how much better our brains and our bodies will work when we are hydrated! I encourage my clients to drink at least half their body weight in ounces of water each day. You may need to drink more if you are sweating a lot or if you are taking any medications that may cause you to urinate more.

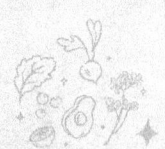

What I ate or drank

How I felt, physically & emotionally, after having it

What I ate or drank

How I felt, physically & emotionally, after having it

What I ate or drank

How I felt, physically & emotionally, after having it

Date: ___ / ___ / ___

What I ate or drank

How I felt, physically & emotionally, after having it

What I ate or drank

How I felt, physically & emotionally, after having it

What I ate or drank

How I felt, physically & emotionally, after having it

Date: ___ / ___ / ___

What I ate or drank

How I felt, physically & emotionally, after having it

What I ate or drank

How I felt, physically & emotionally, after having it

What I ate or drank

How I felt, physically & emotionally, after having it

Date: ___ / ___ / ___

What I ate or drank

How I felt, physically & emotionally, after having it

What I ate or drank

How I felt, physically & emotionally, after having it

What I ate or drank

How I felt, physically & emotionally, after having it

Date: ___ / ___ / ___

What I ate or drank

How I felt, physically & emotionally, after having it

What I ate or drank

How I felt, physically & emotionally, after having it

What I ate or drank

How I felt, physically & emotionally, after having it

Date: ___ / ___ / ___

What I ate or drank

How I felt, physically & emotionally, after having it

What I ate or drank

How I felt, physically & emotionally, after having it

What I ate or drank

How I felt, physically & emotionally, after having it

Date: ___ / ___ / ___

What I ate or drank

How I felt, physically & emotionally, after having it

What I ate or drank

How I felt, physically & emotionally, after having it

What I ate or drank

How I felt, physically & emotionally, after having it

Date: ___ / ___ / ___

TIP #5

Self-care is not just about manicures, pedicures and massages.

It is about filling up your proverbial cup. Feeling whole, refreshed and rejuvenated. Self-care can be different for everyone, but the important thing is to make time to practice self-care every week, if not every day. It doesn't have to be a big event, but a little something each day to remind you that you can and should spend some well-deserved time on you. If you're finding it challenging to practice self-care, try scheduling it into your day planner or online calendar, or finding an accountability partner to help keep you on track.

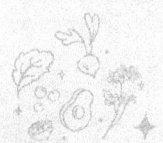

What I ate or drank

How I felt, physically & emotionally, after having it

What I ate or drank

How I felt, physically & emotionally, after having it

What I ate or drank

How I felt, physically & emotionally, after having it

Date: ____ / ____ / ____

What I ate or drank

How I felt, physically & emotionally, after having it

What I ate or drank

How I felt, physically & emotionally, after having it

What I ate or drank

How I felt, physically & emotionally, after having it

Date: ___ / ___ / ___

What I ate or drank

How I felt, physically & emotionally, after having it

What I ate or drank

How I felt, physically & emotionally, after having it

What I ate or drank

How I felt, physically & emotionally, after having it

Date: ____ / ____ / ____

What I ate or drank

How I felt, physically & emotionally, after having it

What I ate or drank

How I felt, physically & emotionally, after having it

What I ate or drank

How I felt, physically & emotionally, after having it

Date: ___ / ___ / ___

What I ate or drank

How I felt, physically & emotionally, after having it

What I ate or drank

How I felt, physically & emotionally, after having it

What I ate or drank

How I felt, physically & emotionally, after having it

Date: ____ / ____ / ____

What I ate or drank

How I felt, physically & emotionally, after having it

What I ate or drank

How I felt, physically & emotionally, after having it

What I ate or drank

How I felt, physically & emotionally, after having it

Date: ___ / ___ / ___

What I ate or drank

How I felt, physically & emotionally, after having it

What I ate or drank

How I felt, physically & emotionally, after having it

What I ate or drank

How I felt, physically & emotionally, after having it

Date: ___ / ___ / ___

TIP #6
Celebrate your wins!

It is so important to celebrate every single day! We often get conditioned by society to keep our wins to ourselves so that we don't come across as showy or egotistical. But celebrating every single day allows us to see that we are wildly capable, worthy and unstoppable! So find one thing to celebrate today. It can be anything big or small or anything in between. It can be a promotion at work, your kid taking their first steps or just getting out of bed when your alarm goes off! Celebrate in your own, unique way and embrace those positive vibes!

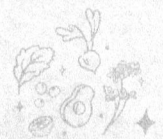

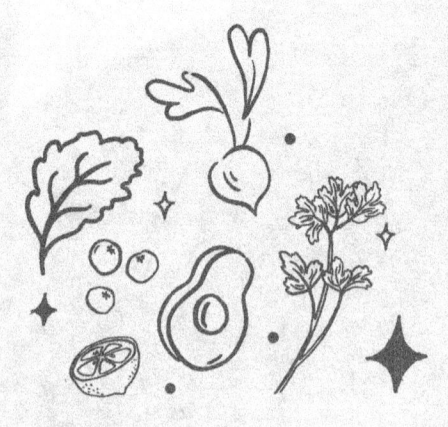

www.ingramcontent.com/pod-product-compliance
Lightning Source LLC
Chambersburg PA
CBHW071844290426
44109CB00017B/1920